Emergence

By Pamela Piatt

DEDICATION

To the doctors who struggled to save me,
and to the entire staff
at Mary Free Bed Rehabilitation Hospital (2013-2014)
I will be forever grateful to you all.

Table Of Contents

Foreword

'Emergence' was a term I first heard from my psychologist at the rehabilitation hospital that I was privileged to be a patient at. A privilege? To be a patient? At a rehabilitation hospital? What is so privileged about that?

For this particular hospital-everything.

I had lost it all. My ability to sit up, lift my arms, walk, feed myself, bathe myself, wipe my own backside, brush my teeth, swallow, breathe deeply or talk loudly or for long periods of time, everything. My memory bank files were officially a wreck and jumbled out onto the floor of my mind. Gone. Everything. Because of two scratches on the back of my neck which let in a staph infection that went septic. It started on my spine and worked its methodical way throughout my body nearly killing me. A motionless shell was all I had left to rebuild with; that, and some of the best therapeutic and hospital staffing personnel in the world that I call friends to this day. They believed in my ability even when I didn't. They found me when I was lost and confused by more than the winding hallways of my new home unable to put the numbers of my room in sequential order let alone match them up to an actual room. They pushed me when I wanted to quit. This, essentially, is their story too.

Pam Piatt 2015

To get started for *Emergence*, we

need to *Journey Back*.

New Home, Fresh Start

*I am awake: So much light, so much activity, ssshhhhh, please. I think I have the equivalent of a medically induced hang over. I feel exceptionally cranky and mean. Ok, low down nasty bad grumpy works as a definition, too. I want a bathe. I want to wash my hair. I want to brush my teeth. I want, I want, I want. And by God, I wanted it yesterday.

   *Spouse is in the room and clucking words of hope and relief, which is for some unknown reason, very annoying to me, I want to tell him to shut up but my trach hole doesn't allow me the privilege. Then there is the fast moving nursing technicians fussing over and around me, checking this and then that, making sure that everything is in its place and doing its proper job. I want to tell them to leave me the hell alone, for pity's sake.

*I can't talk, I can't move, so I cry. Big mistake-I can't hold a tissue to blow my nose either.

*Spouse sees the water works, naturally misinterpreting them, and offers more words of support while he dabs my eyes and wipes my drippy nose which further inflames me. I am not upset at being here! I have a blasted hang over and want to be left alone! Don't open the curtains, draw them tight; the light is too bright on my drugged eyes.

*Judas priest, just shut up and stop trying to 'sell' me on this place and its furnishings as if I 'm picking out an apartment. I'm here. Let it go at that.

*Then, Lord have mercy, some idiot comes in and tells me to smile for the flaming camera…holy moley! Will it never end? I hate my picture taken on my best days and this is definitely not one of those. Much to my chagrin, as I review the results of the photo shoot of the day, I reminded myself of the Star Wars figure Jabba the Hut and I am not exaggerating. Make your way through what I had just endured, and I wager not even the prettiest high priced fashion model would look any better than me on that particular day.

*Thankfully and eventually, the business of settling in settles down.

*As the briefest of time passes, and it is presumed that I am cognitive enough, I am told that I am in my new 'digs'. For how long, no one ventures to tell me. I discover much later that this depends on me and the actual physical progress that I make; progress measured in a rehabilitation type of way. A proverbial ax over my helpless paraplegic head this progress orientated goal is. I would recognize it later as a double edged sword that would cut both ways, in then out through my heart.

*But for the now, I soon get acclimatized to the daily

schedule and expectations of the new home. I am loved.

I am nurtured. Most importantly to me, though, I am

accepted for who I am and not what I can bring to the

table. This is an exciting, exhilarating, and novel concept

for one such as me...

Chapter Two

The

Initial

Days

*My earliest of days in the new homestead are a bit memory blurred what with the brain injury (stroke) that I had endured. Just the salutations and introductions to my first of what would become many roommates was an incredible journey into the frustrating. There was then the seemingly impossible task of trying to learn everyone's name and job description. Then there is the self imposed uncharted path of being on my best social kiss-butt behavior to all the wonderful nursing technicians that I would soon grow to love as my very own. And the social kiss-butt behavior would become real; a smooth integral part of me. Not as before when it was job ordered.

*My initial reaction to all of this wonderful help and nurturing: I hated it. It was extremely difficult to accept, even graciously. From being feed, to being bathed, to being dressed, and having your back side cleaned up (my own particular road block), I hated it. I hated asking for help from already overworked nursing staff, albeit that it was always with a smile on their lips and a song in their heart when they came to do the required task at hand.

*But in real time, when you're use to being the one that everyone looked up to for fixing their wrongs and making things right, it is incredibly humbling and eye opening to be so unbelievably vulnerable for absolutely every need of the human body. How could you even contemplate being grumpy and disillusioned with the 'miracle of life' when someone is happily cleaning your backside up for the zillionth time in a day? It is mindboggling to me. I know that I couldn't have done their job as well or as compassionately; and definitely not without gagging.

Clothes

*I soon learn that I am expected to wear clothes here. What a unique idea after nearly thirty days of being butt naked and covered only by sheets, tubing, and wires. It is all of the everyday usual clothes except for underwear. (Underwear interferes with catheter tubes and big adult diapers.)

*Oh, lovely! I can't move any major flippin' body parts and I am supposed to do what? Not to worry, though. My various technicians had that issue covered; including me and my sorry self in no time. It did not matter that these professionals were a fraction of my body mass. I was twirled, flipped, tossed and dressed before you could say 'Hey you guys....' I had many, many wonderful nursing technicians, male and female but there are two that I affectionately named Thing One and Thing Two, (Becca & Courtney) for their ease of rapid transition in the dressing procedure. I swear they tag teamed me when they had to dress me! It was like a wild, naked ride on a fast roller coaster and I enjoy the memories of those times to this day. Many thanks go out to Dr. Seuss for the foreshadowing of Things to come. For me, it got to where being naked wasn't such a hedonistic behavior and became a breeding ground for comic relief with my extraordinary care givers. I found that it made a normally embarrassing situation quite tolerable, and it helped me to build an exemplarily reputation among staff.

*Believe it or not, this wearing of the street clothes does serve several purposes, though: it frustrates you to no end, gives many people watching you a good belly laugh for the day, and it gets you in the mindset that you will be recovering enough to go home…so help me God.

Side note: If you progress in developing body movement, part of the unique positions you are encouraged to do while dressing is called 'bridging' whereby you are on your back and you lift, or force in my case, your bottom up so that you can pull your pants on. However, I was a muscular weakling and much preferred the excitement and ease of having some help.

Toiletries

*For thirty days in the other hospital, none of these essential items were a part of my life. As a matter of fact brushing my teeth was a horrible three to four minute tasting process of crud on a sponge which was shoved into your mouth and swirled around. (It can remind one of the Biblical reference of when Jesus was on the cross dying and they offered up vinegar on a sponge to him). People kept brushing away at the interior of my mouth in spite of my facial contortions and quiet meditative thoughts of what I'd do with that sponge to them if the positions were reversed; what I'd give to be able to move my arms or even one lone middle finger!

*My various roommates soon brought my senses around to the vast array of fragrance that I had been lacking in the hospitalized setting. The hospital world that I had gotten used to consisted of fragrance free bar soap, baby shampoo, tiny tubes of old tasting generic toothpaste and nondescript lotion. None of which tantalized the numbed senses of a brain and spinal injury patient.

*I was soon exposed to the wild wonderful world of scented deodorant, delicious tasting toothpaste, minty refreshing mouthwash, shampoo and conditioner, exotic smelling foaming bath gels and washes, sleek razors, gallons of scented lotions and body butters, blow dryers, curling irons, pounds of assorted make-up items, which include an easy dozen of different neon colored nail polishes and, of course, nail polish remover, cotton balls, tweezers, and tissues; what hospital stay would be complete without them or be tolerable for patient, nursing tech, therapist, and general population alike! Friends far and near chipped in to make me smell human again. But the products did so much more; I began to be interested in my appearance and presentation, and not just my survival. I was no longer a smelly robotic blob that just existed in limbo.

*Ah, civilization-again.

Pressure Relief

*Pressure ulcers occur when there is too much unrelenting pressure on any one part of the human body. Also commonly known as bed sores in many circles, they are difficult to heal up simply because of what causes them. So if the patient is bedridden and cannot move around for themselves, the only recourse is that staffing must move the patient regularly, often times propping the patient up to maintain a specific position to avoid these sores. They can occur anywhere on the human body if there is pressure cutting off circulation from the living tissue. Some specific sores that can occur are on the head, back, bottom or the legs. I personally experienced some on the back of my head caused from thirty days of being on my back and the continual rubbing of the hard cervical (neck) collar that needed to be worn after the neurosurgery on my spine. My tailbone was red at times but a medicinal cream and eagle eyed nurses (Cherie, Andrea, Tara, & Leslie) kept that at bay. You learn to hold your breath as you are rolled hither and yon, inspected like a fresh vegetable or fruit by nursing staff. They are on a mission to keep you safe and healthy, and sore-free. You let out a sigh of relief when the verdict comes down that all is well (clear) on your naked vast bodily domain.

*Pressure sores resulting in open wound care are a tedious business for a paraplegic and can have extremely serious consequences if not monitored daily. So, to educate (or traumatize) you as a newly made paraplegic patient, they will let you watch ancient DVD's regarding skin care, and pressure reliefs designed for the wheel chair clientele. You are taught the importance of being highly vigilante of your body. I warn you-these videos might come in fading technicolor but the frighteningly horrifying message gets across very clearly, especially when willing RN's tell of their past experiences in other places at other times of diverse patients that grew open pressure sores and the parasitical infections that can happen within the wound. All because the patient didn't think pressure relief breaks were important to their over-all health from the bottom up-literally (Thanks Cherie, I'll never pooh-pooh pressure reliefs again and I m permanently paranoid about my backside!).

*Throughout my stay (until I was able to move myself around in the bed) I was rotated like a chicken on a rotisserie at a neighborhood deli. There are few things more annoying than to finally be asleep in a non-sleeping environment only to be woke up and asked which way you wanted to lay for the next four hours. However, I eventually trained them not ask such a redundant question of me at such an ungodly hour of the morning. Just do something with me-anything, and add pillows for good measure. At that, everybody was happy. And I loved playing one tech against the other when the shift changed occurred during the night. The third shift tech (Selma) would come in with a hearty laugh and a wicked twinkle in her eyes and ask what I was doing with my naked backside openly exposed gleefully mooning her as she started her shift and I would lovingly blame it on the earlier tech (Priscilla, 'popcorn maker extraordinaire') leaving me like that…a patient has to have some fun…not everyone was up on my mobility skills.

*I felt particularly happy and vastly more independent during my stay when I was taught how to scoot up in the bed without assistance, pestering everyone for the umpteenth time. (Thanks Patsy, you are a genius or desperate; probably both!) I still held out for the over-all heave ho with two techs on either side of the bed to hoist my slippery sliding body up in the proper area on the bed.

Thanks bunches to Selma, Terry, Audrey, Hillary, Carlye, and leg shaver-Katye Lynne for always answering my call button, and all of you other great helpers in the early morning hours, forgive my memory lapse. It was early. (And I had had a stroke you know...our own private little joke.)

*So if you ever hear a little beeping sound coming from a wheelchair and then the individual does a peculiar little body shift, chances are you can safely assume that they are doing what is called a 'pressure relief' and that they do not necessarily have body crabs.

Lifts System-Up, Up, & Away...

*My all time favorite piece of equipment in the early days was the patient lift. It was the source of much amusing and breathe stopping entertainment for me and the roommates with and without the nursing staff. Picture if you will a series of metal tracks above you secured to the ceiling that run over the bed area and into the bathroom for each semi private room. Within this manual mobile track is a motorized cable lifting system operated by an electronic controller (with a television-like remote wand) whereby the patient is gently hoisted up, and out of bed, and into power chairs or onto the proverbial commode. The nursing technician must manually push the cocooned patient to the area of choice in the room once the patient is suspended in space. But first, to cocoon the patient, they have to be maneuvered and positioned into a body sling. This is done by flipping the patient from side to side (Becca, Courtney,

Cheyenne, and Shae from the World Wide Wrestling association) and tucking the folded sling underneath the patient. Then the sling is connected in a specific order to the controller so that said patient doesn't fall out of the stupid thing thereby incurring another spinal or brain injury. The body sling is then part of the essential equipment that the patient sits on day in and day out so that there is ease in the lifting process from the beginning to the end of the day. There is a wet sling for the shower and therapeutic pool and then a dry sling for the mundane everyday routines. The endless variety of entertainment that this piece of equipment gave us all was priceless, especially with my creativity still intact.

*This was the most freeing of experiences during my stay, and often times, as I was being hoisted high, I would break out in a variety of song ranging from, "Fly Me to The Moon" or "Somewhere Over The Rainbow", unless the lift was for the commode, then it took every ounce of concentration to focus on bowel control until I reached the landing zone. Techs soon learned not to get me laughing at the essential critical time. If only I could have controlled my own wild imagination, sorry Courtney and Cheyenne, but I did warn you about making me laugh.

Neuropathy

*This is the term given that occurs when there is significant nerve damage and the nerves are not happy about this, so they create havoc and throw hissy fits for the person in the human body. It is usually paired as a symptom of the late onslaught of Type Two diabetes. However, to broaden the scope of occurrence it can occur with any variety of bodily injuries but especially with significant spinal injury. It oft times can mimic the feeling of a burn, a tingle, that sensation of your body part falling asleep, or just plain hurt. To date, my feet, round the clock, feel like they are on fire at different places on them. At one point early on I was brought back to bed from a full day of physical therapy and the very bottom of my feet hurt. It felt just like I had blocks of wood with a grid pattern stuck on the bottom of my feet. I could actually feel the ridges and begged my husband to take them off. (I couldn't sit up yet to view these mysterious blocks for myself.) He looked at me very oddly and then at my feet and swore that there was nothing on them. I continued to beg him anyway. Just then a nurse tech came in and he asked them to verify his accounting of the condition of my feet. She confirmed that there was nothing stuck to the bottom of my feet, and I knew for certain when he began the nightly ritual of lotion and massage for my feet. The pain was immediately excruciating! To this day I suffer from overly sensitive toes with overall feet sensitivity at the end of a long day. Just taking off the compression socks can be extremely painful as one grip's the toe section of the sock and peals them off with a yank. It's kind of like quickly ripping a band-aid off. *A dear and close friend from rehab days (Kyle) suffers horrifically from this condition no matter what the pharmacy can throw at him. Often times he can be seen shaking his hands and tucking them under his arm like a hen protecting her chicks under her wings. In spite of this he is outgoing and friendly and never complains about it. All things considered, he considers himself a very lucky man because he survived.

Spasticity

*Your nerves play a game of 'guess-this-pain-if-you-can'
feeling. I personally have felt three separate types of pain.
One feels like a thin hot poker is going straight down into
the flesh to the bone (internal). Another pain is sharp
needle-like (surface), and the third pain is truly strange. I
can sense a spinning (building) feeling (like an old wind-up
toy) and then it is released when I spasm the closest body
part. For instance, I was in a theater and was very grateful
that no one was sitting in the sit in seat in front of me as I
felt the spirals start up in my foot and then my leg shot up
and hit the chair. Later on at home my hands started
joining in. They will begin to tremor and have a more
severe mild spasm as well (texting on a mobile phone is
perilous as I have sent incomplete messages or woefully
non-illegible words). This proves to be a wonderful excuse
for reaching out and touching someone in a most unsocial

way, especially if they are particularly annoying to you or the populace at large.

*Another character of spasticity is tight or stiff muscles and the inability to control those muscles. I had a wonderful therapist (Mark) who I jokingly called 'Doctor Death' and who came faithfully every morning to do a series of stretches and leg movements. Eventually, with daily consistency, my legs were able to hang freely as I was lifted to and fro in the lift system.

*Even now, though, in comparing notes with my other buddy from that time (Russ) he complains of the stiffness and cramping particularly after sitting to watch a television show or riding in a vehicle for any length of time. I know that even now, as I stand up to do the dishes in the morning, I am stiff but also my legs will spasm and cramp from the feet up. It tends to slow down your response time for running to get the phone or rushing here or there within the confines of your environment. Especially if your

bent over cursing the cramps and gripping the counter

tops.

The Stinky Side of Nursing Care...

*Well, let's discuss what we all truthfully wonder about if we carry certain thoughts to a logical conclusion. Am I the only one to ever wonder about bodily functions when watching a pioneer movie regarding the sick and afflicted? Ok, but let's dialog about this anyway. I love being part of the 21st century and experiencing flush toilets but what do you do when...your body is as responsive as an infant's. Well, they have what are called 'bowel programs' which train your excrement to be ready for a speedy delivery-with a whole lot of help and specific tools. For the average paraplegic this is tantamount to life. One excretes because one will build up with toxins and systems will shut down causing death if one doesn't. But how to do this if there is no feeling to push? Laxatives the night before and plenty of time to relax and let the body do what it must do the next day-early in the day and regularly. Don't try to rush the procedure because it will only backfire on you later. There is also the loving term called digital stimulation. I was threatened with it on several fun filled occasions, and I will not name by who but you know WHO YOU ARE Becca. The technician will partially insert one of their gloved greased fingers up into the anus and wiggle or rotor root the poor body cavity waking it up, stimulating it, and demanding compliance. There are other tools for the sole purpose of scooping (like small shovels) and these are available to aid in the process if the body can't get rid of the pay load. If your mobility is impaired there is a hot dog tong looking tool that, with toilet paper wrapped around the ends, will help for a cleaner more sanitary wipe. One uninformed patient escort confused the assortment of tongs in our bathrooms with barbeque season, "Hey, what the heck is going on in here…"

*Initially though, depending on the condition of the

patient, large disposable pads are placed under the patient to let the good times roll forth or huge diapers; liken as with an infant. However, for urine we have progressed in the health care field. Catheters which are basically tubes going into the pee-pee, drain the urine from the body into a small sometimes premeasured plastic bag. This bag has to be emptied regularly by way of a small valve at the base of the unit. A Foley bag. The catheter (tube) is held in place by a small balloon structure in the bladder which helps to prime the pump so to speak and keeps the urine flowing. There are distinct advantages to having this technology. For instance, if you are lying prone in a bed, not able to get up, (or if you could care less) this technology is wonderful. If you're knocked out for surgery and the team doesn't want pee all over their feet, it's wonderful (even if urine is sterile). In physical therapy though, oh baby. As you are learning to do transfers (with or without a board) this is similar to a medieval torture rack as you are expected to slid from here to there with a smile on your lips and a song in your heart. The rubber tube sticks to clothing or the sitting surface be it exercise mat or wheelchair and pulls against the forces that hold it in place giving the owner all sorts of instantaneous pain (like guys getting hit in the lower free standing groin anatomy). I didn't realize how much this can create havoc until after an excruciating day of practicing sliding transfers, which was accompanied by a wee bit of blood in my Foley at the end of the day. I made my concerns clear the next day in therapy (Mary & Diane-'Sequoia') when I was suspected of being a no good slacker (come on admit). I offered, in my most logical voice, that we try pulling a tube out of their urethra slowly twisting it back and forth like a crazed methodical snake and see how they liked it. I reckon my comment was worth a momentary brainstorm session as my suggestion caused them to think on it, and together we developed new techniques to incorporate into our therapy sessions around 'Ms. Foley' and company.

*When the time comes to graduate and pee on your own it's exciting, exhilarating, and frightening. Now is the time to see if your body remembers how to do what it learned to do and not to do when you were about 2 or 3 years old. The big day arrives and with much sweating and reassurances that pulling a balloon out of your itsy bitsy privates will not hurt, out it comes lickety-split. Mine did not hurt. Others might disagree. (Feel free to have an opinion here.)

*Now, after such a long time not functioning, the medical community has devised a way to be sure you are peeing all of your pee out of the ole bladder when you do pee. They run an ultra sound wand (looks like a smooth upside down ice cream cone thingy)over your lower tummy (bladder) and this measures if and how much pee is left in you. Ever the innovative soul, I imagined the process to be an impregnation device by alien forces which were trying to overtake the planet earth. I would shout out in mock horror as they rolled the wand over my lower tummy shouting out about the abuse that I was enduring. Then I would ask for specific DNA for my alien baby. It made a routine non-evasive procedure fun as I conversed openly about seeing Elvis and Big Foot on the space ship as the rounded magic wand moved over my belly and tried to measure how many embryos were *not* implanted inside of me. As most medical procedures were, this provided fresh fodder for fun with my beloved nursing staff.

*On a more serious not however, for some patients, the work will never end. They will need specialized help to urinate for the rest of their lives. If not totally immobile, single self catheter sets will be counted among their tools of the trade, so to speak.

*They do not feel the need to urinate so they will automatically induce urine flow with the catheter set regularly (approximately every four hours) around the clock. My hats go off to you if you are among this dedicated to life group.

Patient Escort Services

*Now stop chuckling! Stop it right there! I am not referring to the oldest profession business concept that you might think I am. While I was receiving my rehabilitation, these people had the incredible job of knowing the building from top to bottom and sideways. They had memorized the endless trails of stairwells and lonely connecting hallways of the hospital.

*These particular staff are given a schedule of where every patient is supposed to be and at what time. They are cogs of the machinery that keeps all the various schedules running as smoothly as possible. The chain of rehabilitation command is not so complex but if one element of it is off the whole will suffer. It is kind of like throwing a pebble in the pond. Ripple effects are frustrating to a time centered well oiled system. Patient escorts are the 'monkey in the middle' and help to correct any time constraint deficiencies from top to bottom. When patients cannot move, literally, these unique staff personnel keep us going. (Many hospitals are retooling due to building design and staffing cuts but while I was there at this particular facility, the patient escort system was an integral part of the day to day routine.) *Each of my escorts was kind and attentive not only helping to move me through my day but caring for me along the way. I considered them my safety net when out and about during my day. What one couldn't do another could. I am reminded of an instance when I was out cruising in my newly acquired red power chair thinking how independent I was. I was going to check out this place since I had only experienced it from a horizontally confined space…on my back on the hospital bed. I neglected to remember that I had had a stroke and some things were still jiggling around upstairs. Out I headed with smiles and good natured banter from the nursing staff. As I headed into a new to me section of the third ward I realized my oversight as to acknowledging my impaired cognitive abilities…I was lost! Panic seized my gut as my pride rose up. I could figure this out I just knew I could, but the more I went this way and that way the more my rattled brain refused to help me and I was woefully confounded. I tried every method that I had used as a teen in the woods around my home for I was no stranger to survival techniques. I began going over my path methodically, like an injured confused bird in flight. Unbeknownst to me, I was being watched. A patient escort was looking and observing my lack of progress and my sporadic thought pattern. After accessing his paper work he realized that I was on a floor that didn't correspond to my schedule. He quickly and quietly came up to me and asked me where I was going upon which I lost all my stupid pride and vocalized my great disparity. He graciously took me back to my room and at a much later time, we laughed as he recounted his disbelief and self talk watching me through the windows of another floor!

*I later had need of instant mobile intervention from another wonderful patient escort who saved me from a fellow patient stalker by swiftly wheeling me around into an elevator and whisking me to the safety and sanctuary of my own room!

*Thank you to the guardian angels in patient escort. I for one am glad that our lives collided…☺

Chapter Three

Essential

Equipment

Chairs of Wheels

Once you are up and semi functioning, it is determined that you must be fitted for transportation-of some sort. You must travel here and there in the mundane routine of your therapeutic existence so name your insurance company's choice because it will ultimately be your choice as well. There are the ever popular power chairs that go with a push of a small lever forwards or backwards and have zero turn capability. If you make 'connections' with a certain on site wheel chair representative (Paul) he might be able to jazz up your model and make it go just a wee bit faster. At least that's what my dear friend Kyle bragged about. Not being mechanically minded, I could have cared less-until I tried racing with Kyle for free popcorn on Fridays in the open hallway to the cafeteria. But, I digress.

Once up and running (Ha-Ha, paraplegic joke) I was

diagnosed with a left side deficit surprisingly enough *after* I

was fitted with a hot, red, mean looking power chair.

Nothing says midlife crisis quite like a fire engine red model of

anything… I just had this hard time not running into stuff

on my left side, like walls and people. Eventually word got

around about my lack of sweet driving skills, and office

doors would shut when I was 'out and about' with my chair

doing therapy. It was just easier that way; for everybody,

and safer, too.

Eventually, I learned to overcome my left side deficit,

thank you occupational therapy (I love you, Jen), and with

the hard earned ability to sit up (thanks Sequoia-Diane, my

strength) I moved into a less costly model; the everyday

plain old black wheelchair which would take me home. But

even in the non-powered wheelchair arena there are

Volkswagen's (Bugs), Ford's, Chevy's, Chrysler's, Cadillac's, and the ultimate-Ferraris'. I learned to read a person's stage of paraplegia and how long they had been sitting in a 'chair' by the model that they had and their knowledge of it, its maintenance needs, and their dream of next year's better model.

Non-powered chairs, the run of the mill old regulars, can really give you an upper body work out. You learn to appreciate varying terrains such as tile, linoleum, or concrete and groan when you see a stretch of carpet (low shag or not) or turf. Being in a wheel chair puts the rider at times socially in an awkward position. One needs to be aware of one's surroundings always. If you are around smokers and in a chair you could get accidently burned when their hand moves down to their side or another eye opening reality is that your face is level at most people's butt level so if they are talking to you and turn around quickly-oh, boy. I prefer to utilize this moment as a teaching time to the non rider and give them a gentle goose or slap in their posterior parts if I know them well enough-those dog gone spasms…☺

*However, it is vital to learn the safety features of being mobile in your new non-powered wheels. Locking down before standing up is imperative and prevents you from looking like an incredible fool (and feeling like one, too) as you bruise yourself in the worst possible way at the south end of your anatomy, a poor choice for a new injury if you sit on it all day long. This also gives your intuitive therapist something more to work on with you as they will make you get up off of the floor with the same stupid chair without any hope of human intervention (Mary)! Either way a wheel chair means that you have moved along the road of recovery. Something that you didn't think you would ever do. Like the first set of real car keys, so is this, your first set of wheels-connected to your chair.

Side note: A handy accessory to the wheel chair experience

is a pair of the very fashionable sport like gloves designed

to assist the wheelchair user by protecting the hands and

also gripping the wheels more effectively for greater thrust

power when in motion. If you exert less to propel, you can

go farther for the day with less exhaustion setting in.

*I still have mine just in case I want to dress for a special

occasion…☺

The Ever Friendly Amigo Cart

*I choose to place this early piece of equipment among the wheel chairs simply because to me it is the hybrid that offers a different focus of independence balanced between power chair and wheelchair. Some familiar advertising markets label them as a 'Scooter' or 'Amigo' cart and for today's independent mildly handicapped person it is a life support system for shopping in our ever larger, constantly growing, football-stadium sized department stores or warehouses. Prior to my illness, I began using the store offered brand of these devices because my knees were shot to pot. Consequently, I was at a complete advantage when the probability of this tool was offered up on the proverbial serving platter. Initially, I got tired very easily with just a long therapeutic session. Practicing walking with a cane would exhaust me. So, I added this option as well to the menagerie that would come home with me.

*This tool is highly portable and comes in handy for treks out to the garden and around the yard. It is a wonderful babysitting tool as well. The grand girls love to ride with Nana on her go-cart. Nana usually has to take the start up keys out when we arrive at a designated place in the yard and carry them in her pocket or the little stinkers would high jack said cart and leave their Nana far behind as they gleefully ripped up the yard...

Walkers

*I am not necessarily talking about older people at Wal-Mart either…ok, poor joke. These I refer to are the average garden variety types with two basic structures. Surprisingly enough, when my time came in physical therapy, I was scared to learn the nuances of therapy with this particular tool. One is commonly known as the 'cage' walker. This specific type folds in two places to make transport and storage easier. You would see these typically in a nursing home setting but here they are tantamount to a tricycle with trainers. You can't take off, rolling rapidly, in the initial stages of walking if you have to lift or push your 'bird' cage *before* you. You must be able to stand upright and support your body without losing your balance. Balance and strength is practiced continually as well as so many other things within this walking system. You would be surprised how exhausting each stage of therapy is and this one is no exception.

*Eventually you graduate to the world of wheels once more as you and your walker evolve. This next type of walker comes equipped with a seat! Oh, happy day! You walk a bit, and then you can sit a bit. It comes with a braking system like a wheel chair, too. And like a wheel chair, you had better have your brakes on before you plant your bottom or reverse the procedure and stand up. This type of walker is like a wheel chair that the design engineers screwed up on. It is the missing link between chair and cane.

Arm Crutches and Canes

*I had a small child ask me the difference between my 'tools' because she noticed that I would switch them up from Sunday to Sunday. It was a very astute observation from a five year old and I love the fact that she was curious enough to politely ask! Most adults just stare until you notice them gawking. When you smile back, they look away embarrassed; at themselves and at your disability which weighs in on their social caste system.

*An arm crutch is different from a regular crutch in that it does not go under the armpit with the weight of the body resting under the shoulder on it. The arm crutch has a forearm band that encircles the forearm and the weight of the body is distributed via a small handle just below the banding off to the side of the crutch. The band prevents a large diameter of wiggling and jiggling as you try to equalize your weight distribution. It is a very stabilizing tool and when I am in varying natural terrain or when I am extremely tired (dragging my left side a tad) I prefer this over a regular or four footed cane. (I can barely manage my current two feet, adding four more is pushing the envelope!)

*In exploring the world of canes my therapist (Mary) and I tried a four footed model after a stint with a cage walker. I was not impressed with it and neither was she. It was difficult because of the four feet. If you did not actually lift it up and bring it down evenly on those four feet it caused more instability and, consequently, I did not feel safe using it. We immediately switched to a regular cane for the last stretch of my therapy at the rehabilitation hospital and I now use a regular cane even more so, breaking away from the arm crutch except for extreme situations. Like most well used, time tested tools, it is hard to part from the security of these.

Bath Chairs & Over the Toilet Toilets

*Oh, the joys, decisions, and expenses of buying that new furniture you never suspected that you would have to invest in-at least not until you were 85 or 90 years old. Let's begin with the essentials, the ever popular bedside commode (Selma, please stop it...) or a drop arm (not the patient's) commode which fits over the existing plumbing; this was my own personal choice for home and as it came with a free price tag from an earlier donation I said, 'Yes! I'll take it.' It was only in use at the Piatt palace for a relatively brief season but it was a real day maker for the continuous trips. It is currently in storage happily awaiting my joint replacement years. Before I was discharged my OT (occupational therapist-Barb) and my PT (physical therapist-Mary) came to the home to make an inspection of sorts to be sure that necessary doors had been widen, plumbing changed over, and my overall ability to function would not be hindered. We had the plumber replace the original tub with a walk in shower stall prior to my illness thinking that we were making necessary changes for a set of aging parents that might have to live with us never knowing the change would be for me. So, it is within the once master bedroom's bathroom that my shower chair still stands and is used every day. It has delightful suction cups that will annoy you to no end when you try to remove the blasted thing to clean the shower stall. But it is a wonderful invention nonetheless with a grip bar to the side and a non slip surface to sit on so that you don't smash into the fixtures as you scrub your sorry self clean from the day's accumulated by-products. My wonderful PT (Mary) encouraged me not to be rid of it too soon and I have followed her advice given the neuropathy in my feet and the vertigo in my head. We have an assortment of grip bars in the bathrooms as well, and my shower has a removable facet wand to rinse those hard to reach places; like your

face, your back, your arms, your legs, and the nether

regions…

Bed Helps

*While at the rehabilitation hospital, we would practice with these particular tools to be sure that the patient knew safely the 'how to' before leaving for home and hearth. There was a pretend apartment with rooms that mocked up a home. I still sweat bullets as I remember practicing board transfers from a wheel chair to the bed surface. But, as usual, I digress.

* There were two particular tools for the bed. One is a bed rail or bed assist bar and another is a bed ladder.

*The rail is just what it implies. It's 'arms' would go under the mattress and then the patient has an instant rail to help pull themselves up out of or drag themselves onto the bed. I used mine for a while until I couldn't stop getting my feet tangled up in the blasted thing no matter where I put it (sorry Barb!), so I did the next best thing and that was to pull it out from under the mattress and throw it into my clothes closet with a few choice words! In defense of my seemingly irrational behavior a hospital bed's rails at least can be positioned down but this is a stationary rail and will not be moved, unless the mattress is flipped up which I was tempted to do on more than one occasion.

*Next, there is the bed ladder. It is sort of a replica of those fire escape ladders for children's rooms that hang from the escapee window frame. It is a quirky looking thing used to help you pull yourself up or lay yourself down very gently and in

s l o w -m o t i o n. It comes up from the foot of the bed and has rope rungs that help you gradually pull yourself into a sitting position or gently ease yourself down. There is also one that resembles a water skiing handle as well. If there is no mobility from the waist down, this is a great tool for in bed adjustment. In my own creative venue, I had talked with a former roommate (Jayne, look-your name is in print!) at a soft ball game. We compared 'being home rehabilitation notes' and she confessed to using it quite successfully whereby I asked her if she enjoyed water skiing off the bed in an upright vertical position. I had an immense laugh and so did she as we envisioned her standing up on the foot of her bed and riding the waves in a two piece little bit of nothing…Yee-ha!

Dressing Tools

*This subject leads us into my own personal purgatory; compression hose-ouch! Initially at the rehab hospital they had used compression hose to reduce the fluid build-up in my lower legs. My wise nurse tech (Patsy to the rescue again!) monitored my legs religiously. One night while preparing for bed, I became aware that the back of my leg behind the knee was hurting; right where the hose had been pulled up to. Upon inspection Patsy noted a pressure abrasion from the tight hose. That was enough for me. Until we could find a pair of hose properly suited for my personal needs I refused to wear them. As I have stated before, pressure sores are to be avoided at all costs. The back and forth concerns of the day were discussed with me regarding the on-going swelling of my legs and feet. This was not something that would go away. Eventually my OT Barb and the supply coordinator found a brand with a medium compression rate that worked.

*Now let me lay out a mental visual for you. Donning compression hose is like trying to put a spandex body suit on a wild greased pig; I don't care how skinny you are. I've seen experienced nurses and techs alike brace themselves with fortitude when it came to the vicious tug of war that compression hose presents; especially if your patient can not help you in any way such as keeping the leg stiff and ram rod like. During my hose-less leg period I would watch one of my roommates put on hers. She was paralyzed from the mid-chest cavity down, and worked like a dog to maintain her leg position, body balance, and pull those things on. The first time it took her twenty minutes for one leg! I was fascinated at her perseverance (way to go Megan!).

So when my time came to add compression hose to my ensemble, I was not a happy camper. But OT (yea, Barb!)

to the rescue! There is a variety of dressing aides but particularly for compression hose (dah, ya think!). In home health care equipment, there are many different types of tools for the same purpose but it is an individual's choice to select what they feel comfortable with. I choose a tool that resembles a PVC pipe cut in half and flanged on one end. There are two holes on each side, and strong boat-like rope that is attached through the holes. You thread the sock on to the non-flanged end then, in a sitting position, you put your foot into this tube of sorts and pull the sock on over your foot with the rope. Adjustments are then made and an overall inspection of the hose is done to be sure there are no wrinkles (particularly around the ankles) that might cause pressure sores. Perfecto! Ready to roll!

*Getting your shoes on and off is little better than donning the hose. Many people just switch it up to do the Velcro strap foot wear but ever the tight wad that I am I had a really nice expensive pair of shoes I had bought prior to my illness and so I began laying the floor plans to be able to use them-by myself. After all, the key to rehabilitation is to become as independent as possible and I was determined. OT to the rescue again-Barb! There are elastic shoelaces that are laced and tied up once) if you do it right) and then you can slip your foot into the shoe. The elasticized shoelace also helps to 'give' for the swelling of your feet at the end of the day. I was very weak at this stage so Barb developed and sewed on the tongues of my shoes loops so that I could use a hook like dressing tool to pull on the tongue while sliding the foot in. There are also very long shoe horns for the patient who stands to put on their foot wear and this of course keeps the back of the shoe from curling up causing one to curse profusely particularly if you are running late…joke.

Just a side note: During my outpatient stint I told my OT

Barb about my inability to load my left foot and leg into the passenger side of our vehicle. Try as I might it was a frustrating challenge and exhausted me. I lost all desire to even go for a ride because of it. So, she created a large sling of sturdy fabric that I could drop under my foot when seated and efficiently lift my leg and foot up into the passenger side of our vehicle! It is in my car to this day.

Grabbers

*Oh, the wonderful world of reaching out and touching someone, but I digress…again.

*This is a tool that was developed originally, I think, for short people. Now, don't go getting all huffy and politically correct on me…I am short (5'3") compared to some. I have learned to deal with it and so should you.

*Grabbers were developed to avoid having a dislocated disc or a hissy fit which results in elevated blood pressure prior to a brain bleed (i.e. a stroke) for the average type person-handicapped or not.

*This is a long handled tool with bug like pinchers on the end controlled by the squeezable handles on the other end.

*To operate you first locate the item you need (up above or down below) put the pinchers around the desired item, squeeze the handles which make the pinchers close around the selected item, and abracadabra, you have your heart's desire on the end of bug pinchers! I have used my grabbers to reach cereal, to plug in my computer (under the desk), and to put the Christmas tree skirt around the base of the tree! I have used one set of grabbers to reach for other grabbers that fell out of reach! I have used them for items above my head and for items below my waist at floor level. You can get expensive booted up models that are liken to a Swiss army knife with gee-gaws and whistles, or the plastic plain Jane's at the dollar store.

Chapter Four

Speech Therapy

Tumbled Thoughts &

Scattered Shot Sound

*Some patients don't know *why* they are scheduled for speech therapy, and grumble as they have to wait in the queue for their allotted time slot. I for one *knew* why I had to have this very specialized assist. I could barely make a sound (hard to believe, I know) upon the day of my arrival at the rehabilitation hospital not just because of the tracheotomy hole in my neck but also due to the fact that my rib muscles in a conspiracy with my lungs had not had to work very hard for approximately two and a half weeks as I was on a ventilator in ICU. To make matters worse, the infection had made every part of my functioning body weak beyond belief as my system fought death.

*Speech therapy obviously deals with the ability to make recognizable language specific sound but it also begins at the starting point of the brain where the need to communicate and reason originates. I am a stroke patient. I have a spinal injury. I was *screwed*…

*So began the approximate five month journey I made with Lindsey, my beloved speech therapist, to reorganize my thought process, develop my lung capacity, and consequently begin to communicate with the world around me once more; this would alleviate my frustration and society's. Essentially, it also began the rebuilding of my cognitive processes to prepare me for the work force once more. I am eternally humbled and grateful to you Lindsey, though I never vocalized it to you: you, the very one who helped me to find my voice…

*It all started with inhaling into a little plastic contraption that had three differently colored blue balls confined in separate tubes: a spirometer. The object was to inhale enough to raise those blasted blue balls to the top of their tube homes and, later on, to hold them there. Sounds easy enough, right? Not with limited air supply, or the lack of ability to produce said air supply. The nursing staff (particularly Nancy and Leslie) was in cahoots with her, too.

"Have you done your puffer today, Pam?

"How many repetitions did you do today, Pam?"

"Now don't make that face at me Pam."

"Here, I'll put it on your bed tray so you can reach it, Pam"

"Oh, it's no trouble at all for me Pam. I'll stand here and count for you as you puff Pam."

"You know this will help you not to get pneumonia and make you stronger Pam."

"How did you know I was going to ask you about it Pam?"

There were smirky smiles by both contestants in this dialog battle.

*To add insult to injury, Lindsey, bless her heart, set me up with another type of tube puffer thing that hung around your head like a cheap dramatic dollar store necklace. This way you could turn eight shades of red as you puffed away on it in public proving to all that you were not negligent in the ever progressing fight to improve your lung capacity at any available chance you got!

*A chain smoker had nothing over on me…

*As much as I fought the exercise, it did indeed help me on my way to be able to say two and three syllable words once more without stopping for a breathe in between. It also developed my ability to speak in more than just a whisper. However, I kept going hoarse with my newfound voice and testing had to be done to ensure that there had been no damage to the vocal cords during my ICU stay due to three tubes that were down my throat at the same time. The continuing coughing mucus flare ups, in spite of medication, didn't help either. So I got to have this delightful little test whereby they stick a tiny camera down your throat beyond the uvula and then ask you to talk so they can see the vocal cords in action. After trying to cooperate and not get rid of my last four meals all over everyone, it was decided that there was no permanent damage done and it was merely extreme inflammation causing my problem. So, I was ordered to give my vocal cords a rest-except for speech therapy-by speaking in whispers and absolutely no singing or loud vocalized screwing around. This would prove a harrowing delicate social balance for me and for Lindsey as I loved to sing in my lift systems, pool time or otherwise; and then there was my exuberant zest for life and a rousing good joke. If not brought in check, I would be totally hoarse by the time speech therapy rolled around making her job virtually impossible. So, I was on strict orders from my firm 90 pound soaking weight speech therapist from singing or even talking loudly, preferably not at all. Call me paranoid but I think it's kind of a shady call-come on, speech therapy and I'm not allowed to practicing my sweet new skill? This doesn't seem logical to even me-a stroke patient...☺

*She emailed my physical therapist (Mary) and together they negated my 'stroke' card excuse to keep me on the straight and narrow. Sigh. I was a problem patient.

*The other aspect of my rehabilitation that speech therapy worked on was my cognitive recognition, skill in repetition, and memory, as well as, the skill in verbally communicating it all back. This would prove easy at first as we narrowed down my therapy needs. I could remember words for time lapsed recall but figuring out complex interpretive pictures was quite another matter as you had to relate and project possible scenarios using logical deductive reasoning; my mind was stretched to perform. I struggled to find a voice for the words that I could see but was at a loss as to how to pronounce. I am still slow in communication if stressed to verbalize a specific thought or need. The right word will sometimes escape me as it drains out of the word closet of my mind. Or I will see it and feel it but not be able to say it. Both occurrences are equally frustrating.

*Particular games over word search puzzles proved to be harder. Learning basic math skills with an addition concept was easy but subtraction and any real life story problem that would use this concept was, and still is, a challenge to me. Eventually, I would learn to use a keyboard again slowly incorporating it with computer software preparing me for my return back to the work field.

* Flash cards in math and clock faces to stimulate the brain, and 'as loud and as long as you can say aaahhhhhh' sessions may have grown wearisome but the results are wonderful.

*It was all incredibly difficult and tiring day after day, month after month. The advances seem miniscule when you are on the trail to life once more, but looking back, I

find an immense pride and accomplishment as to how far I

have come from where I began. I not only had physical

handicaps to work through and overcome but the mental

handicap proved just as exhausting to rise above; it

uniquely tied into myself worth as a contributing member

of society and ultimately my internalized self esteem.

Chapter Five

Occupational

Therapy

Occupational Therapy: For the Everyday Experience

*Oh, the ponderously frustrating joy of occupational therapy. As in all types of therapy, this one, too, is designed to push the patient to the performance max-in the everyday rubber-hits-the-road format. Occupational therapists are there to prepare you to go back out into the non-hospital world with an unappreciated level of ability to brainstorm yourself out of any sorry situation. It's the question of 'What matters to you?' versus, 'What's the matter with you?' And how are we going to get you there.

Two therapists and their OT's in training stand out in my mind: Barb and Jennifer, and their respective students, Jessica and Stacey, who were at the hospital at the same time I was fulfilling their required fieldwork.

*When I was admitted into the rehabilitation hospital, I was a tetra-plegia more commonly known as a quadriplegia, where I lost the total use of my limbs and torso. Paraplegia is similar but does not affect the arms. The loss is usually sensory and motor, which means that both control and sensation are lost. My spine was not severed so it was a matter of let's wait and see. In the mean time they would put me through my paces. Initially, I had a lot of swelling due to the damaged kidneys so the initial response was to put my hands in a rather elegant pair of tight fitting spandex type gloves and when I was in bed I was to have my arms propped up above the level of my body. It was rather like being in a soft fluffy body cast. Eventually, Jess would make a hard plastic cradle for my arms to keep them straight at night and annoy the heck out of me.

*She would gently wash my arms and massage lotion on the arms and hands to stimulate the blood flow and help loosen the muscles. Soon we would work on specific exercises always taking it just one step further and farther, meticulously every day. If I was her I would have gone berserk over the slow snail like progress that we made. Washing my face was a big deal as she rinsed the washcloth in very warm water and handed it to me. It felt wonderful to put it to my face and know how much pressure *I* wanted to apply to my face. Brushing the teeth would follow and was quite a sticky messy affair at first. There would be the old emesis basin and two cups of water, and lots of towels! I had difficulty hanging on to the toothbrush so Jess cut to fit a spongy tube over the end of the handle and I was in business! I needed her help squeezing the toothpaste on the brush but when it came my turn to try I quickly learned to squeeze the toothpaste down into the bristles of the brush so that it wouldn't fall off before I even got it to my mouth! She slowly began to build other toileting skills such as brushing my hair (we needed to be careful because I had bedsores on my head) putting on deodorant, and the big laugh of the day-trying to get enough strength up to push and twist into a bra. With her patience and persistence I was able to learn how to do all the basics all over again. All of this was done with her bedside and me in the bed because I couldn't even sit up on my own yet.

*(The nursing technicians would have to feed me early on in my recovery rehabilitation process until I regained enough mobility and strength to manage the task myself.)

*I first wrote with Jess. Down in the therapy gym I asked if I could write my name. I do believe she was stunned. No one had suggested it up to this point. Excitedly she fetched paper and pen. I wrote first to my husband. Then I wrote a thank you note to a dear friend who had organized and ran a fund raiser for me in my community back home. I was beyond exhausted after writing these. Handling a pen and forming thoughts in a comprehensive fashion may not seem like a tiring muscle pumper but it is after a stroke and paralysis.

*Some of us on the floor needed additional helps and so the OT's were constantly tweaking methods, trying this and then that, to help each of us reach our goal of independence. Part of my later needs with Barb would be truly life alternating (at least for me). Barb would brave the wonderful world of culinary delights and get me back up to speed in the kitchen without endangering myself or the world population at large. She developed more individual tweaks for me and totally equipped me for life out in the 'normal' world. More importantly, she made me think situations through to figure out a safe and probable answer for any handicapped situation. Rolling into a variety of bathrooms and making practice transfers onto the stools was a nerve racking session for me. I began to realize how important building code was to the handicapped person right down to the way the door swings on the stalls. Thanks to my OT's, I can tell you just by the look of a room if a person in a wheelchair is going to be able to effectively maneuver within said rooms or certain public building environments. I will never again complain about the expense of handicap building codes and neither would you if you had had my experience.

*During my out-patient therapy time, Barb and I fine tuned any areas that had not been covered during my actual hospitalization. This included elastic shoelaces, a loop to help me get my tired gimpy leg into the car, and practicing how to get a full backpack on and then off as I had mentioned my desire to go back to college. We also practiced putting my walker in the back of the car and taking it out. At that time I doubted that I would ever have the strength to go out into public alone as I was so exhausted just preparing for the event!

*Jennifer and Stacey were not to be undone. I had a variety of regular board games and torturous cognitive proofing games to do. There was also a big electric board on the wall that would blink and you had to be quick and push buttons for responses…this worked very well for getting responses out of my beloved OT's, too.

*Jen had the extreme pleasure to help out one day by putting me into my bathing suit for the therapy pool. It was needless to say a good deal of fun for me as poor Jen turned eight shades red and perspired profusely turning me this way and that pushing and pulling the suit on my uncooperative wiggly body. I laugh as I remember her face to this day! She has more than likely blocked it from her subconscious.

*Jen also introduced me back to the world of the World Wide Web computer life. I had lost most of my stored information regarding my email accounts and so we reestablished me into cyber space and took a stroll through her favorite place on the internet at that time-Pinterest. ☺

*All of my OT's had prepared me from dressing, to toileting, to cooking, to laundry, instilling me with bravery and confidence for the new world I was about to step into. Yours is a uniquely noble and honorable profession. May you never lose the hope that you so effortlessly pour into the patients you serve and who so desperately need you to light the way out of the everyday darkness of despair.

Chapter Six

Physical Therapy

The Essential Element: Physical Therapy

'A long time ago in a galaxy far, far away....'

*I could sit and I could walk; *without a wheelchair, without a
walker, without arm crutches, and without a cane*...that was then
and this was my now. I would have to learn to do what I
had *naturally* done in my infancy and toddlerhood at the
ripe old age of...well, never you mind.

*I was to be given the unique privilege of learning how to
do all of this again from, literally, the ground up; but on
this journey I would be accompanied by an even more

unique person fully equipped for the task at hand: Mary (Marium). (Later, I would affectionately call her Marilyn as in Monroe).

*She had in her quiver a band of merry men (women) just like Robin Hood. There was Diane (Sequoia, my rock), and Jess of physical therapy fame (not to be confused with Jess from occupational therapy-do you sense my frustration at keeping everyone straight? After all-*I had had a stroke-right Mary?*), and occasionally Jacalyn and Rita when scheduling was a factor.

*The first annoying thing about Mary was her attitude. It was always, and I mean always, upbeat and positive. And she was *never* at a loss to incorporate my failures into a therapeutic session. No matter what I threw at her. Eventually, she would learn that I could be trained relatively easily by waving an occasional Hershey's chocolate kiss in front of my nose or thrown into my waiting mouth like a seal. I am sure she would say that I barked about the chocolate loud and long enough…☺

*She was also in cahoots with my rehabilitation doctor (Dr. Ho). At team meetings (when they discuss your case without you being there) I am certain that she reported on my infinite lack of progress, lousy attitude, and my unfailing excuse making. Yes, she was a difficult obstacle to overcome but I was determined. ☺

*I do not recall my initial meeting with Mary. It is as if she and I have always been a therapeutic team with her holding the harness (and the whip ☺). We would spend nearly five months together and then roughly an additional three months for outpatient therapy. Her guidance and immense patience with a very difficult patient is why I can live an abundant life today totally ambulatory and productive. She would humbly say that God had a lot to do with it as well, and I would wholeheartedly agree with her.

*With speech therapy working the cognitive and lung strengthening, the occupational therapists working my fine motor skills adapting to current abilities, physical therapy would begin to rebuild my large muscle strength and promote viable use. (For every day a patient spends in bed horizontal, they lose weeks of muscle strength so I had a very long way to go.)

*My original prognosis from ICU was not a good one. It was projected that I would spend the rest of my limited days on this earth unable to be conscious of my surroundings, and if I was conscious I would be unable to communicate with anyone and so I would live in the back room of a nursing home on kidney dialysis fighting infections and bed sores until death released my body.

*Well, surprise, surprise, surprise! I did wake up, and though my brain files were tossed all over the floor of my mind, I was very much aware of my surroundings and as my speech therapist and physical therapist can attest, I was not going to be a quiet placid patient content to wallow in martyrdom.

*Prior to my designated time frame with physical therapy which was each and every day, Sunday through Saturday, my legs were stretched. We were then rolled down to the gym and lined up like the waiting, blushing debutantes that we were, gossiping about everything and complaining viciously over the hospital board of fare (food). Each of us was fighting off the nervousness of failure in that gym; in front of everyone but particularly in front of ourselves. I cannot express adequately or completely the vulnerability that you have as a patient in this environment. You struggle to rebuild yourself physically, internalizing this incredible situation emotionally, and it causes you to analyze your spirituality, or lack thereof. At least for me this was true.

*Begin at the beginning, and I did. I needed to get my natural balance back-finding my core balance. Within the confines of the wheelchair and bed my body found comfort and support naturally. Now I had to find it without those tools. And so began the adventure for Mary and Sequoia. Mary realized that this was not a one therapist job so enters Diane (Sequoia). She earned this nickname from me because of this aspect of therapy that I needed to acquire. Now, you might think that this is really a redundant idea to have to learn to be able to sit up without the benefit of any environmental tools but it is harder than you can possibly imagine. I have a whole new respect for babies and all that they have to learn now.

*It began by me being placed on the mat via lift

system…and being held in place. This exercise is all about strength and a feel type of thing. Mary and Diane told me that I learned it very quickly. In only about three or four days I had figured it out. Mary would put me in a sitting position standing in front of me, Diane would be behind me with pillows. She was to catch me in a puff of pillows when I lost my balance and fell backwards. Remember I had little if any arm and hand strength so supporting myself in that way was a no go. We worked and worked for an hour a day. Mary sat me up and Diane would count seconds out loud noting how long I could stay upright. After a particularly grueling episode, I lay against Diane panting for air and laughing. Suddenly it just popped into my mind (as most stuff did back then) the picture postcards I remembered as a kid with the car driving through the middle of the redwood tree. I immediately claimed her to be my Sequoia redwood tree, there for all ages, encompassing the area and supporting all the wildlife (which was me)☺.

* With this lesson intact and well learned I was able to move on to more arduous tasks. One of these was being able to transfer from surface to surface. At first you learn how to use a board as a bridging surface. Hence-a board transfer. This sounds easy, too. But it can be downright dangerous if not done properly. You place the transfer board under your thigh to cover the handle hole on that side of the board than place the other half of the board on the surface you wish to get to like a chair, or car seat, or bed making sure that the other handle hole is placed on the desired area. When all is secured you simply slide over to the board to the designated spot. You remove the board from the underside of your opposite thigh and ta-da! You are moved to another perch without any assistance.

*And so Mary and I began to rebuild this 'Frankenstein'. My left side did not want to cooperate with her or me. In the early days as I lay in my hospital bed at night I would force my limbs to wiggle. I would stare them down and try mind over matter. The big toes first because I could see them from this angle, then I tried flexing a calf muscle, flexing anything. I needed something to give me the courage and inspiration I knew I needed to face the next day of unrelenting therapies. I would break into tears as I failed in the attempt letting the disappointing rain fall down my temples into the pillows and sniffing so that I wouldn't need a nurse to wipe my nose and consequently see my shame. Silly, I know, but real for me nonetheless.

*Slowly my right side began to lead the way. Without leaving my wheelchair I was rolled in front of machines that specialized in upper body exercises and then rolled in front of machines that specialized in leg building. With my legs strapped onto foot pedals, I began to pedal my way back to regain the strength and the memory in the left side. Still it was not enough.

*I slowly developed a way to move my legs at night. Initially, I worked on my right side as it was a willing partner. I would move the toes vigorously in every direction I could think of, visualizing the anatomy of the leg the whole time. I worked up the leg by flexing the calf, thigh and then shift my butt muscles to move the hip thereby having the effect of moving the leg. It so encouraged me I began focusing on the left side. This proved frustrating. From the tip of my toes to the top of my thighs my legs were as dead. But my butt muscles were intact and I would shift and flex them, slowly I was able to move the leg using the hip! I am not a genius. I was desperate. All of the team work of all the therapy working together gave me the shot in the arm my body and mind needed. Let's face it-what else did I have to do besides wait in the darkness with my irrational night time anxiety until the morning shift came on to begin another day. *Ever so slowly Mary took me through every trick in her physical therapy book. Still it just wasn't enough…

* I would be fitted for leg braces. Great. Deflated balloon. I had seen a variety of leg braces parade back and forth in the gym before me and I was not impressed. It brought back childhood memories of polio victims consigned to a life of clanging metal and slapping leather with off balanced walking towing arm crutches to the sides. I had been hoping to avoid this for myself. Nope. A hideous pair of white Velcro strap shoes was bought and the braces were attached with much measuring and adjustment of the bolts. Frankenstein arrives at the ball in full regalia.

*I was to try out my leg braces with the walking frame. Not

only did I officially look like Frankenstein with those puppies on but I could barely walk due to my lack of mobility. Hence enters the walking frame. It is literally a sturdy metal frame with handles and 'arms' to rest your forearms on, you hang on to and it supports your entire body weight as you concentrate on moving forward and utilizing the legs. It was my first time moving in an upright vertical position since my illness. The late night experiments with my butt and hips came in handy now. I threw my weight from side to side via the hips and slowly ever so slowly forced that damn frame forward. Family members there cheered. Mary and Diane cheered. Fellow patients cheered. I sweated like a bull moose in heat. I went about ten feet that day, it seemed like a good long country mile. This would take forever if that's all I could accomplish in one thin therapy hour!

*Dr. Ho wanted more as well and faster, too; the last of the remaining tricks in his bag-The Pool.

*I love the water even if I do swim like a rock. But the nervousness I felt as three therapists prepared to get me into the chloride laden graduated three to six foot depth water developed into something far greater and more overwhelming.

*And I was being loaded in by a ceiling lift system. Now don't get me wrong-I loved my lift system in my room, but it didn't have water under it and I could always Marine crawl on the floor without drowning. I was reaching a whole new level of terror as I was strapped into the water lift hoist. I shook and not from excitement. Had I come this far through so much to only go out by drowning? I put on a brave face and hide my unease in wise cracks. They had to know. But they hide it beautifully and encouraged me every step of the way. As I was lowered down with unmovable feet dangling I dropped gracefully and slowly into the warm shallow water. I felt the warmth as my left foot went under first. I wiggled my toes! They moved! My whole left leg kicked and responded to my muscle commands as I relished in the warmth of the water! It was as if I had never ever been paralyzed! As my body sank into the water I forgot my fear. With three therapists around me I moved my entire leg length and shouted for joy. I was a crazed mermaid. They couldn't talk either, but Mary, Diane, and Jess had the biggest smiles on their faces and just shook their heads yes as I screamed, "My leg is moving-I can move it! I can move them both-look, look you guys!" For the first time in months I had true hope. I choked back my tears of joy and in the gravity reduced environment began my true recovery and strength building regime. Loving arms helped me to stand for the first time in months and as I gripped the pool parallel bars, I began my journey back into the world of walking.

*The next time in *my* pool, and for all the many times after I would sing as I was lifted high above the water and gently lowered in. I would walk in between parallel bars and go from shallow to deep ends focusing on gait and balance exercises in the warm life giving water.

*After the progress in the pool my land locked exercises became more challenging as we tried to replicate the pool successes onto dry land. This would be sweat producing hard work.

*My strength returned very slowly at first as was evident in the exhaustion I felt each and every night after therapy. It became a joke on the floor between my fellow patients and me that I was in bed by 7:30 and not to be bothered with their shenanigans. Usually I was up and ready to go by two or three in the a.m. but no one seemed to appreciate my sense of humor at this unearthly hour except for my roommate Jayne and our loyal nurse technicians.

*My life developed slowly around the physical schedule of therapy and as my transitional countdown time to leaving the hospital came closer we started working on floor transfers. (I can see Mary grimacing now…) They like to make you practice getting up off of the floor by yourself just in case you have the stupidity to get there on your own to begin with. And this is a good thing…

*I was terrified as I saw a team, a whole team, of black uniformed clad PT's coming at us one day with nervous smiles slapped on their faces and Mary was giving me all the false hope that she could muster. This will be good she said. You've got this she said. I'm gonna let you try this on your own she said. I was not comforted.

*The first thing I learned how to do the hard way was the

value of letting yourself down *gently* to the ground surface. And I had an exercise mat under me.

*The tricky part for me was my blasted arthritic bone-on-bone knees. This was another reason for the pool and the anti-gravity environment. So we all sat on the floor together while I thought about my predicament. They waited and just smiled…

*I tried this way and then I tried that way avoiding my knees at all cost. Blast it to smithereens. This was a virtual impossibility.

*Initially I knew that my upper and lower body strength was limited and I had to make each effort count. I tried sliding backwards to the elevated mat but my arms would not lift me up that way no matter how much I cursed and sweated. With no option left open to me, I rolled over on my poor knees. I began to pull my way up onto the mat in a belly down stance starting to feel quite smug. But I started to flounder-big time. My strength was officially gone in my upper body and I began to slid down off the edge of the mat. Instantly with much verbal encouragement and great muscular gung-ho four PT's picked up about 75% of my dead body weight and slide me facedown-tummy down unto the elevated mat. They felt quite accomplished I'm sure getting my lifeless bulk off the floor without a portable lift! I was laughing so hard I could not help one iota and when they had deposited me on top of the mat they were laughing and sweating in unison with me. They privately acknowledged that they could never remember a more non-professional transfer in their combined lengthy careers. All in all I think it only took about 20 minutes. Needless to say, I did do better later on with my burgeoning endurance.

*There's this vertical table with a real technical name that I forget now-I chose to call it the lobotomy table. It looks like something out of a science fiction mad doctor laboratory movie. For the unskilled eye it resembles a regular old gurney or examination table. But it has straps along its entire length and can be slowly positioned in an upright vertical position. When you first start to stand upright after a lengthy horizontal position or even a long term sitting position your body can get mixed up on what it is suppose to do for you as far as regulating blood pressure and heart rate. A quick drop of these can cause you to pass out without the ingesting of any alcohol.

*I watched the patients. I watched the therapists as they monitored the stats. No one threw up but there were lots of pasty faces after wards. How hard can this be I wondered. Silly naive fool that I was; my turn came. The idea is to get the back side of your body as close to the surface of the table while they strap you in. My knees revolted. My stats were fine, my head was fine, and my stomach was not sick but my knees were killing me because one the straps that had to be tightened were right at ground zero on top of the knee. As Mary tightened the straps around my knees, I thought I was going to pass out-from the pain. But as usual I sucked it up and grimaced for about 20 seconds as the table was elevated. Let it never be said that I was a non-cooperative patient! Grumbling and sassy maybe but I always tried when put to the test. This exercise did not last long and I eyed said table with contempt from that moment forward. But lest I grow slack in my need to straighten and improve my walking posture there was another piece of equipment that was a gentler version outfitted with a seat for brief periods of rest. This particular machine, side by side to a mirror, taught me how I *actually* looked compared to how I *thought* I looked as I stood. Comparatively, they were two very different things and prompted me out of my cocky comfort zone taking walking to the next level that of posture.

*Day in and day out, in a 'one room school house' therapeutic environment, I watched, learned, and worked. For nearly five months I would work just to get to outpatient status. As I progressed, the bitter sweet realization that is typical to therapy became evident. I was working myself out of the very place I had grown to love and felt safe in. I would have to leave my beloved nest and finish the flight of life on my own.

*There would be no soft fluffy pillows to encase me or capture me, no one would answer the call button when a need was on the horizon, and there would be no cheering, encouraging crowd of witnesses to relish in my accomplishments. I would soon have to learn to catch myself, cheer myself, and push myself all by myself. This is the final frontier of recovery.

Chapter Seven

Recreational Therapy

Recreational Therapy

If you didn't know how to live recreationally before, they'll show you how to do it now with a smile on their lips and a song in their hearts.

*This was an aspect of therapy that took me by surprise. Prior to my infection I was a workaholic. Needless to say with eleven homeschooled children and a part time job my life was pretty full. So, I really didn't have time to indulge myself in any of my favorite pastimes which included maniac reading of any genre, a world coin collection, creative cooking and canning, recipe writing, calligraphy design art, and the occasional crocheting project. Truth be told, I hadn't been able to do much of anything for myself for many years.

*As I was wheeled into the recreational department, I was

dumbfounded when asked, "So, Pam, what do you like to do?"

"Uh, what do you mean?"

"Well, you know, what did you do when you were home for fun, like a hobby?"

*What? I can't move hardly any part of my anatomy and you wanna know what I like to do? I would like to walk and get back to my work filled life that's what I wanna do! I naturally remained silent on this point.

*So, I quietly responded with an ancient hobbies list and took an internal meditation regarding my former life style.

*The therapists where very good with me, and very patient. We finally got it narrowed down to calligraphy and then eventually, crocheting. Something that I thought would never be a part of my life again due to my lack of upper body strength and eye hand coordination not to mention my impaired cognitive ability.

*There was always something fun and different going on in the 'rec' room. It was a wonderful change of pace from the traditional therapies that I was receiving. It was laid back and relaxed as we explored just what our bodies could do on a creative level. This core of people was responsible for taking us out in public, equipment and all, to area restaurants and gently helping us find the courage to explore the *regular everyday social stuff* that we had forgotten about in the flurry of crisis, pain, doctors, wheelchairs, and therapy. I was given the opportunity to even do woodworking! I am proud to say that my floral arrangement is beautiful in my wooden planter, and the birds made my day when the bird house was finally hung up off our patio and residence was committed to! As I shed my equipment, these take home projects are wonderful reminders to me of a quieter time and that I can do anything if I try because I did them when I was supposed to be unable to.

*Kelly is one of the most enthusiastic, compassionate, marvelous women I have ever met and she helped to run this department. Kelly herself is handicapped, a rather obvious fact as she rolls around in her light weight framed chair. I became aware that I was not doomed no matter what the prognosis for my recovery to a lackluster life of homebound handicapped-ism after meeting her. She opened my eyes to the world of possibilities as big as the huge picture of her in a kayak displayed in the hallway to the recreational department (at least it was when I was there). There is a vast arena of activity for the handicapped athletes called adaptive sports. They help an individual develop and participate in all varieties and levels of sports such as, hockey, basketball, and (winter) skiing. It is incredible what is out there. Adaptive bicycles, or hand cycles for adults and children are available as well so that they can participate in solid physical activity. There is no need to remain inactive if your health is stable and you have the *heart* for it.

*Other fun things planned for the patients were card or game night via this department. They were the social connect for us all and paved the way for us to interact once more with the populace away from the disabilities that held us so captive. Various nights to create special seasonal gifts for our families were offered. And they brought in therapy dogs to inter react with us. This was a nice break from the sterile hospital setting and reminded many of us of our lives before suffering the debilitating reasons for being there.

*Recreational therapy also provided peer group support night that was initiated with take-out food that *was not on the hospital menu* because it came from the local restaurants in the area! This alone was enough to tempt even the very shiest patient to participate. Real pizza, soft drinks of your choice, sub sandwiches, Mexican, or Chinese was way better than what the hospital could offer just because it wasn't hospital!

*Peer group support night *is* necessary for the newly handicapped. There are the inevitable questions and confusing emotions which become a part of your waking nightmare and you are too shy or embarrassed to talk to the doctors or nursing staff. Let's face it they haven't been there. *(Except one doctor that I personally know of who was called in to address my weird bed sore issues on my head. Unbeknownst to me, she had been called in after I had voiced my concerns regarding my hair loss due to the bedsores I had had. My scalp had a plastic-y feel in areas of my head too.*

I was tooling around the corner and headed down my hallway to get to my room when I came upon a woman walking very carefully and methodically with a cane close to the wall. Initially thinking that she was a patient, I noticed that she was looking around at the room numbers. I slowed down and asked her if she needed any help! Silly me! No she was there to visit a patient. I rolled into my room and she stopped to look at the room number and strolled right in behind me! At the end of our medical conference she felt free to tell me that she herself had been a patient there after a terrible skiing accident that broke her spine. She had to learn to walk all over again! I gained more hope over that one medical consult than the many hours of therapy that I had put in and it had nothing to do with my hair or head.)

*So back to peer support group night...Difficult questions regarding health maintenance out of the hospital setting, marriage issues due to the catastrophic occurrences, family adjustments with or without children, lack of sex or loss of technique, insurance battles (auto accidents), and fighting varying levels of depression because of the whole ball of wax. No topic was sacred and all topics were important. Above all, it has the sanctity and privilege like that of a confessional to a parishioner or doctor to patient. It is a survivor's discussion and is not open for review or judgment. It is a private club and the membership price is a high one, indeed.

*It was the subtle preparation for the last stage of recovery…real life.

Chapter Eight

The Gang

&

Some Fun

"And a good time was had by all…"

*Let us remember that into each life a little rain must fall. I also contend that the sun usually comes out-after the rain…

*Once settled into a not so very atypical routine, the rehabilitation hospital offers a unique environment to establish a social pecking order, at least when I was in residence I found this to be true and it was a life saver emotionally and mentally. You are sharing with total strangers (staff and other patients alike) the most catastrophic health happening of your incredibly vulnerable life whether you like it or not. Semi private rooms are not semi anything in the midst of bathing, toileting, and eating, and medical need. On the flip side of that argument for private rooms I offer this. If it hadn't been for my first roommate (Lois) I would have been traumatized beyond belief as I was new to the world of paralysis and suffered PTSD from my near death existence in the form of extreme night time anxiety and claustrophobia. I not only needed medical attention but I had no way of pushing my call button to summon help for myself. Imagine my great relief in the long night hours whimpering like the frightened pup that I was, unable to move and then to hear the comforting sound of another compassionate human being saying to me, "It's okay honey. I pushed my call button for you. They'll be here soon."

I could only respond with a whispered, 'Thanks.' starring into the shrinking darkness of the ceiling above.

*I developed friendships with each of my seven roommates. And I am happy to say that I was pleased to do the same for each of them when they were new and frightened as well. One of my roommates was moved into my room due to issues with another patient and was not only unable to move but could not speak. I became ready friends with her large family and was able to call the nurses one night when her coughing sounded lose and suspicious to my mother ears. Consequently, she was able to receive medical care and suctioning immediately. Another dear roommate friend of mine was placed with me after a near fatal coding from surgery. She too cried out in her sleep and I summoned nurses as well for her.

*I understand the need for private rooms yet see and sense the need for the semi private in a rehabilitation setting. On this issue, I will say that I was thankful for the hospital setting that I had when I needed it the most.

* The friendships earned and made via the room system

was good for me and I maintain a particularly close bond to this day with Jayne. She too was a transfer due to patient personality conflict and tended to be fairly laid back finding humor in nearly everything. I shall never forget her consistent 3:00am need to relieve herself. One night I awoke to Jayne and our nurse technician Selma quietly singing Madonna's 'Like A Virgin' giggling maniacally so as not to wake me up. Needless to say I enjoyed it all, and we were bladder bound from that point on. It was party time every morning at three and Selma and Audrey were usually our go to girls.

Later on they would decorate the outside of our door like the pediatric ward would do. We acquired the hard earned title of the Princess Room. Jayne was Princess Pee as she had to laugh as often as I did but with far deadlier results.

*Just outside the familiarity of our private boudoir would

be the rest of the floor. One side was for the spinal injury patients and the other was for brain injury. During the run of the mill day with the therapy gym and the comings and goings of our lives we struck up friendships that I shall carry with me for the rest of my life. They know my struggles because these were their struggles too.

*We had a tight knit pool group (John & Russell) with which we exchanged and hurled insults when ever our wheel chairs or paths would cross. I became Flipper because of my obnoxious splashing about and after this heat provoking chide was tossed after me I promptly named the bully Chewbacca (Star Wars) because he was so hairy. I greeted the other one day in the therapy gym loudly proclaiming that I didn't recognize him with his clothes on…sweet memories.

*Our other buddy in the clan was younger than us but he

became my wheel chair racing partner in crime and inside informational guide about the cafeteria. He was so appalled that I had lived so long and never had imbibed a Red Bull energy drink that he felt he had to right the situation immediately. Down we tooled to the gift store racing in the main hallway. I began to wonder if this was such a hot idea when I realized that we would actually enter the gift store in our power chairs and I wasn't that accomplished at operating mine and gift stores are notoriously small and chic with lots of breakable stuff at ground level. Before I could voice my concerns Kyle told me to follow him and in we rolled. Around the back to the south end cooler we headed. He opened the door and pulled out a cold one. He twirled around and paid for it then I followed him out into the hallway. Like two naughty kids he handed it to me and said, 'Here, try this. You're gonna love it.' I had heard so many stories about Red Bull from my own children and those on the floor that I was curious about this poison, so down the hatch it went and Kyle was right-I loved it! The flavor was unlike anything I had ever had particularly in the last few months. So, proud of this accomplishment, I immediately headed back to my room to see how much laundry money I had left in my purse. Enough. Just enough. Back we went for one more! I chugged that baby down and man, oh, man did I soar through therapy that afternoon. I was a bright and shining star! I told certain ones along the way what I had done. They registered concern and asked how I was feeling. 'I feel great!' was my very enthusiastic response. After an hour or two it was time to roll back to the third floor and I noticed a slight headache setting in. As they prepared me for evening stats wrapping the blood pressure cuff around my arm and waiting for the final read out, I chatted uncontrollably. Then there was a gasp. Not from me, from the nurse. Let's just say it was…elevated. She preceded to question me about the events of the day and nearly stroked out when I told her that I had drank two energy drinks in the afternoon. I proceeded to get the lecture of my life from some one more adept at it than my mom. I truly was unaware of the physical changes that occur within the human body after drinking just *one of these cans*. It was lucky for me, and her, that I didn't have any more money for a quick run to the gift shop.

Thank you, thank you, thank you Kyle. No regrets here!

*And when was somebody going to tell me about the free popcorn in the cafeteria on Friday night?

* Kyle was lazily munching on real movie theatre tasting popcorn before dinner one night. I rolled along side of him sniffing like the old blood hound that I was. In a hospital setting your nose adjusts *rapidly* to smells that are *not* of the

hospital environment.

"Dang it, Kyle! Where did you get that?" My saliva was pouring forth like the mighty Mississippi.

"They got free popcorn in the cafeteria on Fridays."

"Well, when were you gonna tell me?"

"I thought you knew!"

"Let's go see if there's any left."

*So off we went down the hallway to the elevators.

"We'd better hurry before they close."

*We revved it up and swung in through the doors. Still open but the popcorn had been cleaned out! Gone! All gone! I had learned a very vital lesson about popcorn on Friday night. The following Friday and for many to follow we enjoyed as many of those pathetically small bags of popcorn as we could. We looked fit for a safari as popcorn overflowed from pinched fingers and stuffed wheelchair bags trekking back to third floor with a faint buttery scent trailing behind us.

*The wheel chair races were rampant on every conceivable social level. Because many of us couldn't stand, staffing had to weigh the wheel chairs the night before the following day. So if you know the weight of the chair then when the patient is weighed sitting in it the next day you just have to do a little subtraction. This was a necessary procedure.

*You knew weigh in day was nearly upon you when your ears could make out the muffled squeals of excitement from late-late night staff in the early-early morning. Straining your ears you could just hear the whirl of soft wheel chair tires on the slick hallway floors around about- well, it was early. When techs were called for bathroom needs, the tale-tell signs of racing would be glistening on their brows as they struggled to breathe in a normal regulated pace whilst answering a call light. ☺

*We patients (well, alright, Kyle and I) had our own version of this wonderful heart pumping past time. There were no real rules other than not letting hospital staffers catch you at it. My favorite hallway was the long segmented run to the cafeteria. Kyle egged me on as we tried to see who could get to the doorway first. He always beat me and then berated my power chair which wasn't nearly as big as his. He hinted around that maybe I could get Paul to make some modifications for speed but I already went fast enough for my taste. When I graduated to my non-powered wheel chair Kyle and I developed a chair train to accommodate our need for speed. I would roll in front of his chair and he would elevate his legs to protrude in front of him making contact with my back and slowly increase speed. It worked out great until I realized that I couldn't steer to make corners or avoid walls very well, let alone people.

*He was a willing shuttle service as well. I caught a nurse tech getting a ride back from the laundry room on the back of his chair! It was better than a golf cart and they only needed to hitch a ride to their designated work area.

*Hospital gurneys are a blast as well under speed and the sensation is totally different in a horizontal position. It can play havoc with your vertigo though, when you look up and see the lights and tiles go zipping backwards.

*I had to have an MRI during my stay but my favorite experience was when I had to go down to X-Ray for some pictures of my knee joints because of the pain on the 'lobotomy' table. X-Ray was located across from the therapy gym back then, and with a sheet over my body-my entire body (yes, including my head) I moaned loudly and gave a few seasoned staffers a near coronary as a talking

corpse was not usually seen in the rehabilitation hospital.

*Great times, indeed. ☺

*Recreational therapists had some planned activities for us

and they were lots of fun but eventually we found a deck of

cards and went from there…

*There was quite a group of us collected around the table

one night out of sheer boredom. Let's face it. you can only

watch so much cable television before you go ga-ga with

the re-runs.

*So, there we were clustered and ready for action, any

action that we could come up with. I don't even remember

the card game that we started but it was a flippin' scream of

tear emitting laughter. One older gentleman in a wheel

chair who had suffered a severe motorcycle accident was

attended by his faithful card playing wife. Due to his

traumatic brain injury he was there only in spirit, or so we thought. He was rolled in tightly to my husband's side as we gathered at the big table. We all very politely tried to include him in on the moving conversation from the card game. And as we became more involved so did he; with my husband's cards. He kept reaching for them and trying to ingest them. My husband kept pulling them back, discreetly of course. Slyly the old gent waited for just the right moment: when we were all distracted by the game. He quietly reached over to my husband's side and picked up a card from his pile. Slowly and methodically he raised the stolen card to his waiting mouth. My poor husband was at a loss as to know what to do or how to handle this delicate social mishap.

*He turned to this man's wife and mentioned that it appeared like her husband wanted to join in the game. When she realized what was happening she cursed her husband loudly (with a sailor-like vengeance) and grabbed the wet card from her husband's dripping mouth. It was all we could do to keep from busting out laughing as she had not been aware what he had been trying to do this for over a half an hour. All of us had been watching the struggle and his prominent success. Occupational therapy was obviously working for him!

*After the verbal butt chewing she inflicted on him, she then proceeded to wipe his drooling mouth with a tissue. The tissue would not stay put on her lap and in exasperation she put it on the table within her reach for his needs. Now he had a new focal point to zero in on and Kyle began watching him in earnest.

*With a few more turns and the inevitable distraction of the game, he went for the tissue. Kyle saw it first as the game had become quite involved by now. Loudly Kyle proclaimed, 'What the hell? Jesus Christ, now he's eating the Kleenex!'

*I noted that this is what hospital food will do to you.

*With a shriek and a new volley of obscene language she jumped up and dug the tissue from her husband's mouth. I could stand it no longer. I absolutely had to belly laugh and so did everyone else, to the point where I believe Jayne nearly wet her pants.

*The wife, too, relaxed and joined in for she found herself among understanding friends who could love and not judge bizarre behavior. Somehow when you've been to the brink of the edge nothing is abnormal anymore.

*On the slow weekends with no scheduled visits from family members we would sit outside our rooms in the hallway after supper as if we were sitting on the front porch of our homes. We would shoot the breeze and gossip about each other and share our wishes, dreams, and desires but never our fears. Our fears were our own private demons and we were in the struggle of our lives to find our lives and what our handicaps would call on us to rise up to.

*And the nagging question always there in the back of our minds-could we?

Chapter Nine

The

Psychological

Factor

My Beloved Shrink

*Alright, no wise cracks. But I must confess that she had
an impossible job before her.

*I was privileged to have a wonderful Doctor to help with
my scrambled brains, or rather to help un-scrambled my
brains and get use to being in this weird state of disability.
She would also consol my spouse into merging into the
same pathway as I was traveling now. This would include
the everyday acceptance of my newly found handicapped
state and the deeper aspects of life. She was a wheel

144

greaser; not an easy task on any playing field.

* Initially, we did the surface stuff. Who are you? What do you do? What makes you tick? Then we got into the fundamentals of our everyday life, discussing how *all* aspects of life with my disability would affect us even though I had not yet come home.

*She nearly had a fit when we explained the severity of the illness and what the choices had been. These were horrific choices that no one should have to make; the pressures from outside forces and certain medical staffers to give up on me, literally-to pull the plug, gave her an insight into what my spouse had had to endure. The obstacles before us would be larger than life. We had met those challenges before in ICU.

*And so we talked, and talked. Eventually, I alone would meet with her for my remaining sessions. We covered a vast array of issues and I found that those memories of our friendship (*friendship to me anyway*) would sustain me in the trials that I would yet face during my time away from the safe environmental cocoon which was the hospital.

*During the first traumatic year of my time at home, when I was particularly stressed I would wrap the gifted shawl, that had been hers during a health crisis, over me at night and cry myself to sleep my fingers entwined in the large loops of soft yarn. Her counsel gave me the strength to press on via the memories we had made though I felt so very all alone.

* Because of her unique counsel and supportive strength in my initial stay there, I was able to come through the blackest of my rehabilitation nightmare. This time comes when you are alone-on your own 'and nothing, no nothing is going right' in the words of artist James Taylor.

The

Doctors

Dr. Samson Ho

*I have had many doctors throughout my illness and my subsequent recovery. The one I came to grow closest to is Dr. Samson Ho. I do not know how he was contacted about my case other than the fact that, when asked where to put me when I came through the worst of my life threatening experience, my husband requested Mary Free Bed Rehabilitation Hospital for any possible therapy that I might be able to do. Little did any of us know at the time that it would be the turning point of my life in so many ways.

*I discovered that Dr. Ho is a quiet, spiritual man early on in my rehabilitation process. He was often times late doing his hospital rounds and this would prove instrumental to me in my acknowledgment and acceptance of my condition and the subsequent limitations for the future.

*The reality of my predicament, the illness, the memory flashbacks, would over whelm me particularly in the evenings when I did not have to be preoccupied with the daytime therapy. Late one night visiting with my husband our talk centered on the freakishness of my spinal infection, the stroke and how horribly painful it must have been. I remarked that I wished I could have some remembrance of it all in order to make it more *real* to me. In spite of my present circumstances, I just could not wrap my head around the fact that this actually *happened to me*. I remarked that it was probably a good thing that I wasn't conscious because of the great pain I must have been in. Unbeknownst to either of us, Dr. Ho had been at the door of my room preparing to enter and had heard my ending statement.

*We turned and greeted him inviting him into our private alcove. I will never forget his commanding continence as he stood at the foot of my bed. As if my current lack of mobility wasn't enough proof for me, he looked very deeply into my eyes and said that he had seen my initial charts and that if I could survive *that* than *Someone* (and he pointed upward) wanted me here. And yes, I should be thankful that I do not remember the pain because it would have been great indeed. I grew very internally quiet at his commanding uncompromised authority as he gently touched the tips of my toes while imparting this truth to me.

*Before leaving us that night, he left me with this mind boggling thought which would haunt, and ultimately fuel my drive in therapeutic recovery, much later.

*"I tell you this now that people who have what you have

had do not live. *Someone* wanted you here, now." His quiet silent authority spoke volumes to me then and even now as it resonates in my memory of that time.

*He silently let me know that I had been given a very special and valuable gift of life with this one simple faith statement. Consequently, I was compelled to ask myself how I would use this specific gift for the rest of my journey here. These reflective thoughts that he gave conception to back then influence my choices of the everyday now.

* Much later, approximately two years later, he would confess to me in a follow up office visit that when presented with my case he wasn't sure if he even wanted to take me on. I thank God now that he did.

Someone wanted me in your care Dr. Ho. You, too, made the right choice in the matter of this patient case file. Let my sincere thank you for your decision ring out; for my thank you will never be loud enough or long enough for your generosity. I will try to do your faith in *Someone* justice

for the rest of my days.

*Doctor Winestone. My neurologist.

*In the beginning of this whole horrific occurrence, there was a neurologist who supported my husband with the difficult choices that medical science laid out on the buffet table of choices. Reviewing my case, he presented my husband with a prominent pulsating life line by passing beyond all of the negative odds. If *she is to live*- she needs the abscess removed. She needs surgery. No matter what the prognosis, *if she is to live* stuck in my husband's ears.

*Do it. Whatever it takes.

*There is a chance that she won't survive surgery.

*Do it.

*Papers were signed. Lots of papers.

*I was prepped for surgery.

*When the majority of all the others were shaking their

heads with the most negative of prognosis's for a very deathly ill woman who, by the way, did not have a lick of health insurance-he stood out from the rest. He was willing to fight for life. He stood above the rest. He gave life a chance. No matter what. He did not push my husband to one decision or the other-*he supported him.*

*Doctor Winestone and I became intimate on an operating table. He did his job well. I am fused at C5-6 and I live.

*Months later I would get to meet this man face to face in my follow up office visit with him. I was verbal and conscious now.

*I nearly tore the place a part, or at least the doors within the office confines because I was sent by special transport to my appointment in my power chair and left side deficit; I had not quite mastered either one of those obstacles yet. Before he entered, I hear him stop outside the door in order to look at the patient file that had been placed in the pocket holder on the door. Within seconds, he bursts in with a total look of surprise on his face and says to me, "You shouldn't be here!"

* I am confused. I think I got sent to the wrong doctor on the right day or something.

I pathetically ask, "Ah, I was told I had an appointment with you today. They sent me here. Ah, which doctor are you?" I had, after all, been dying and unconscious at our first meeting. This put me at a definite disadvantage.

*He then got very excited and talked rapidly. He never knew if I had made it out-alive. He was excited that I was in a local rehabilitation hospital. We compared notes and I updated him on my therapeutic goals. He brought in a young interning colleague and began discussing the miraculous recovery of me. No one on staff had expected me to live beyond the surgery and if I did the prognosis was grim for my quality of life. He positively glowed as he looked at me. He had given birth. I once again had a sharp, professional, defining image of the seriousness of my illness.

*He couldn't wait for my next appointment to compare my recovery in rehab with the current me.

*My next appointment with him, found me in a regular wheel chair and just starting the relearning of my walking skills. I was not yet skilled in this endeavor so the chair was a good traveling option. In my usual independent way, I neglected to wear the very confining soft neck brace which *I was suppose to wear daily*, as prescribed by him. At the end of our brief and happy rendition of my therapy, he looked deeply into my eyes and with a twinkle in his said, "Oh, by the way-you can stop wearing the soft collar now." I left the office room door intact this time with only a subtle scratch.

*Rolling in from the appointment, many of the staff asked

how it went and we chatted about the weather. My loving nurse tech (Becca) nearly had a fit when I rolled by her not wearing my collar for the neurologist's appointment. After a loving chew from her, I let her know that my appointment went well and just before I left his office Doctor Winestone had released me from the offending thing. So there.

*The staff had a heck of time keeping me true to my doctor orders regarding this piece of equipment. This would, in future, alleviate a lot of their stress with making me compliant to doctor orders.

*At the time for my last visit with him, I was still in my wheelchair as I did not have an endless supply of energy for outings. However, I was walking for real in therapy and reported this to him. He was ecstatic and true to his exuberance-glowed. When the office visit was done, he asked very humbly if he could share my smile with some others of his staff. I felt so undeserving but readily agreed.

All of his staff came to wish me well and see the woman

who, with their boss's help, survived the worst possible

odds. I hope they appreciate working for him as much as I

appreciate being one of his many patients.

*He saw me at my deathly worse. Dying. My kidneys were shutting down under the strain of the sepsis and the drugs being used to kill it; hopefully, before it killed me. They were crying out in pain looking for solace and relief from the impossible job set before them. They knew their job but were being poisoned from within. They were battered in the storm for the fight for life.

*Enters the renal doctor. He reads the reports and analyzes the damage. He senses my kidney's needs through the forth coming lab reports. They are shutting down under the strain of it all. They are incurring damage beyond repair. Everything, all of it, will be for naught if something is not done soon.

*Emergency dialysis is ordered up in the hopes of helping the kidneys survive the strain. Those necessary life filters are tiring fast. I am prepped once more. This time a cut of about three inches is made high on my inner right thigh. I am plugged in. During the process I am in such terrible pain that I actually come out of my drugged comatose state and my bedraggled brain was trying to make crazy sense of it all while enduring the cure. I think it is my anal tubes that are pinching and twisted, but maybe it was the incision. I do not know. I just want this burning to stop. I turn to beg for them to stop, please stop, but my voice does not come out. Tubes are everywhere in my mouth. I feel hot tears coursing down the sides of my face. I see red. Tubes of red. I sense people in the room. No one hears me. No one knows of the anguish I am in. No one cares to see. I am a job. No one helps me out of this vortex of pain. Memory intact. These will be nightmares for later, when I am safe in another hospital.

*A year later I have a follow up appointment with another

life giver, my renal specialist, Doctor James Visser. I have been home from the rehab hospital for approximately three months by this time. After about five months of intensive residential therapeutic care and two months of outpatient therapy, I find that I am shy once more when meeting a man of medicine that knew me when. What do you say to a doctor who you don't remember yet helped, as a team, to save your life? I walk into my appointment supported only by my cane now. I am upright and tubeless, I can talk, I can look him in the eye, I have real clothes on, and my hair is growing back and styled. A far cry from what he last saw-

*Stunned. He is surprised. He is astonished. He explains my lab results and gives a plan of care.

*"Your kidneys are coming back. You are a moderate Stage Three CKD. I'd like to see if they come back more." He explains what that means to me in terms I understand.

"Do I have to stay on that awful renal diet?"

"No, but no ibuprofen products. I want to see you back in a year. Let's see what happens in a year."

*And then the statement that I repeatedly hear again and again from the professionals in my life, 'you're a miracle, you know.'

*We chat about my life and how I am doing; back to work, driving, cooking and cleaning; the whole nine yards. However, confession is good for the soul they say, so I admit that I get tired easily. I have to pace myself you know. I'm thinking about some more PT for endurance and strength.

*I do not want to burden him with my depression or feelings of frustration as I go about trying to do that everyday life stuff.

*'Keep it up. I'll see you in a year. You are a miracle.'

*Wow. I am uncomfortable now being elevated so high for I know what it is like to fall from the heights of life.

Epilogue

I am on the other side of this painful chapter of my life now. I have learned so many valuable life lessons that had evidently slipped through my surface grasp previously and I was judged worthy to be slowly re-taught all of the important, deeper, things of this life. I am honored that I was found worthy of the providential effort. I was a good student. I learned and I shall not forget.

I shall not forget the value of human life and the dignity that it demands no matter how debilitated or lifeless it may appear on the outside. Rest assured, the human spirit does exist from within. I know this for certain now.

However, I am glad that it has come to an end. The work was exhausting and the lessons abrasive. I am a complete, lopsided, full-circle back to me.

This I do know. I was never alone. In the still darkness of catastrophic illness and the deeper regions of coma, I was never alone. While I literally slept through the valley of the shadow of death, providential plans were made on my behalf, my long five month journey of recovery thirty days away was already laid out and waiting for me on the other side. Hand-picked individuals going about their jobs in the health care fields of rehabilitation were placed years before I would need them. I believe that every person that cared for me was selected especially for me and me for them, by God.

The canvas of recovery has changed now in the once familiar environment that I woke up in, and many have moved on to change career goals or further their present ones but I know without a doubt that they were there for me because of a much higher power involved. So, together this is our story. I dedicate it to them.

Appendix

No. This is not a body part that can wreak havoc on a person if it gets cranky or blows a gasket. This is part of the subject matter that I want to include in this book. It deals with thankfulness and gratitude.

Many of my medical care providers worked part time hours with little to no long term benefits. This is an unfortunate side effect in the battle against rising medical costs. And yet, these were the people who, not only touched my body, but also touched my heart and soul with their loving inter-personal care giving skills. They were not afraid to get down and get dirty, literally, and most importantly to me, get real. They kept it real. Everything about your new life is initially surreal and frightening. They help you to put it into perspective. They show you how to laugh over your life challenges and kept pumping you up to keep going, to keep achieving even while they might be struggling in their lives just to make the next bill.

So, when I got cognitive enough and farther along in my therapy to do some self searching, I decided to write some letters.

I wrote to the ICU nurses who cared for me and who, for the life of me, I can't remember even though they kept me clean and feed, and perpetually watched me and my precarious condition like hawks during the most unstable of my time.

I also went back, when I was able to walk with a cane, and do a victory lap through ICU and saw my room that I battled for my life in. This was very surreal, indeed. A few were there that remembered my case and specifically me. I was a far cry from what they remembered. I was in civilian clothes and no pipe line tubing in any of my orifices'. It was magical.

The other letter I wrote was to the best world class

rehabilitation team at that time on the planet. These people keep you focused and know when to push and when to let you cry-because they silently cry with you. They know the effort it takes and the mind set needed to accomplish even the smallest of goals.

The last letter was the very hardest one of all to write.

When I arrived, I was in the ugly duckling stage not quite hatched; and I woke up and saw my new family. They loved me by caring for my every need unconditionally. I probably drove them all nuts but they never showed it. This letter would be my Swan Song to them. I was done. I would be leaving the nest permanently and never see many of them again. It was heart wrenching emotionally and I felt actual physical pain over it.

In our technological society I am able to keep in touch via social media but it is not the same.

I have grown up. I have grown away. I walk on my own

now...

March 6, 2014

To the Staff of Spectrum Health (Butterworth Campus) ICU,

Allow me to properly introduce myself to you: My name is Pamela M. Piatt and I am so pleased to finally make your acquaintance!

You may recall 'me' as I came into your lives as a patient on September 8, 2013 late in the evening fresh from the emergency room. My body was wracked with a staph infection which had gone septic. Within hours of a single day, my family was told to prepare themselves-I was not expected to live, not once were they told, not twice, but several times. My physical body began the tiring process of 'shutting down' as a myriad of doctors began the fight that would eventually lead to my recovery. You all were part of this success story. From those that washed my sickened body to those that scrubbed the floor beneath me; you all are a part of me now.

You supported my husband (who kind of looked like Santa Claus complete with beard and long hair), my children (I have 11, yes 11!) and some of the dearest friends a human can ever have on this earth. I thank you for your kindness on my behalf to them. Making a horrific situation more manageable, more wise-decision worthy for them was no less than your quiet diligent care of me. I am so pleased that you were all there to represent me to them. They needed me to be there and I just wasn't able to be at that time.

So, I thank you. From the bottom of my heart, thank you. These are two of the smallest words I know, and they do not represent my soul encompassing gratitude to the best ICU staff in my mid-west Michigan community.

To close this letter of appreciation, I would like to encourage each and every one of you not to ever, ever give up hope in the status of your patients. When in your care, we are more often than not voiceless; nearly bodiless, somewhere between here and there. Please continue to give the quality of care that comes up from the bottom of your soul that would be what you would want for yourself or your loved ones if you had to depend on others to be your hands, feet, and heart.

After leaving the ICU, I was escorted to Mary Free Bed and checked in there on October 4, 2013. I began the slow and tedious process of learning how to swallow (I still love red hospital Jello ☺), to sit up, to get dressed, to wash myself, to toilet myself, to tell time, to figure out where I was in the rehabilitation hospital, to operate a power chair without sending any innocent bystanders to ER ☺, to power my own manual wheel chair, overcoming vertigo to stand (initially in the therapy pool), and walk with various assistive devices such as: leg braces (AFO's) a cage walker, a regular walker, and more recently a forearm crutch to last week's practice of a regular old cane. I felt just as proud at my great old age passing my driver's education rehab as I did when I first started driving at age 15. Thousands of exercises have been done from a variety of specialized therapists. It has been tiring for me as well as them. I am still a bit wobbly and need the support of those around me but none of this would have been possible if you had not been there first and foremost in the most professional medical way to assist me in the job of healing. Thank you. Never stop caring. Never stop performing at your very best peak of quality.

I have been re-instated in my previous job. It is to run the finances and statistical work of the largest private human resource in my county. You have done so much more than help me. Your touch has reached beyond me to help thousands of others that I come into contact with.

And so we are, like ripples in a pond, touching the shores of each. May your ripples be kind, gentle and always shimmering reflecting the light...
Ever Grateful,
Pamela M. Piatt

May, 2014

To all of the Therapeutic Staff at MFB, and particularly to:

Mary, Barb, Jess, and Jen,

You are all my therapists. Each of you is because you are all part of a larger complete circle of professionalism working together for the sake of the patient. You daily redesign and scope out the patient's path of independence and health, helping them to achieve the sought after goal.

I have watched you all for hours on end. Quietly and patiently working day in and day out cheering on even the smallest gain. You, above all else, know exactly what it took to accomplish that very small gain. You also understand the fear, the hurt and the disappointment that we must live with. You understand our great despair when we cannot reach up and out of ourselves to give you, our best and most loved audience, 100% of everything we have left at the end of a long tiring illness.

For it all, the long, bone weary work days that you so very graciously put in, thank you.

Never lose sight of what drew you into this sacred professional career route: It is the patient. When all the insane bureaucracy and politics of hospital seem to take the joy away from your marrow, remember: the patient. You are the patient's only life line towards viable independence amidst it all. You are needed. You are integral in the healing process. You are all special, kind, loving individuals and I count myself blessed to have known you and worked with you.

Again, thank you.
I shall miss you all,

Pamela M. Piatt

May 2014

To all of the nursing, technical, and support staff of MFB:

It has been a few months since I have been discharged from MFB (2/12/14) and soon I will be closing out my outpatient time as well. I have found it very difficult to put into coherent words my extreme heart-felt feelings that I have for each and every one of you.

You provided me with a safe, warm, loving environment that I immerged from a life threatening illness with which left more than just physical scarring and disability. To be truthful, I wasn't so sure I wanted to come back to life and yet as with so many of life's choices I had no other option but to push forward. You all kept the pathway well lighted and defined for me. Often times literally pushing me forward or just finding me and keeping me on the straight and narrow! ☺

I will not say goodbye. It is too painful. But know that my best wishes and thoughts go with each and every one of you as you continue on your individual journeys.

I am glad that our paths crossed if even but once in my life. I can only hope that

Providence will see to it that our paths will meet again under pleasanter circumstances for us all.
Again, thank you for your loving kindness, and all of the fun and laughter...it was the best medicine of all.
Forever and For Always,
Pam Piatt

Pam Piatt 2015

www.ingramcontent.com/pod-product-compliance
Lightning Source LLC
Chambersburg PA
CBHW051912170526
45168CB00001B/356